Stop Smoking 7day

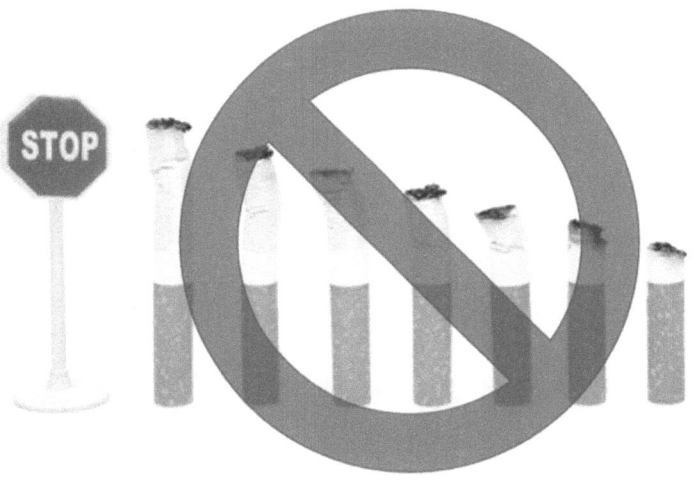

Stop Smoking 7days

Stop smoking 7 days
Copyright © 2012
ISBN # 978-1-105-45671-8
Library of Congress PCN # 2012901458
Printed in the USA
Chicago, IL.

Author - Becky Gruber
Cover Design - Becky Gruber

Research / References – WebMD
Merriam Webster Dictionary – Wikipedia

Becky Gruber
http://stopsmoking7days.info
http://kickhabit7days.com

Index

Introduction

Question: Do you smoke because you like to smoke, or because you are addicted and cannot stop? This is a bit of a trick question. Whatever the answer is, it appears as if you have entertained the idea of going smoke free? "Ha, not a chance," says your taste buds. – "Please do," say your lungs – "Eating more will cause you to smoke less," said your stomach. "Try the patch," says your television – "Substitute your cigarette for our drug," said the pharmacy or your doctor. STOP! You can quit smoking without any of these substitutions in 7days – All you need is a made-up mind and a determination to kick that habit once and for all without replacing it with another bad habit. "Oh yeah, come on, let's do this," says your life. "

If you are like a million of others, you have probably tried to quit smoking once if not several times. Yet, you are still smoking. Regardless if this is your first time searching for a stop smoking program, guide, technique or many times, it stops here. Rather, your smoke intake consists of seven cigarettes a day or seventy; you <u>can</u> stop smoking for good. Cigarette smoking is nothing more than a habitual daily pattern that you can alter. You can overcome any obstacle in life, including years of smoking.

You can and will be successful if you are truly ready to quit.

Stop Smoking Timeline: 7days

About this book

Finally, a totally FREE way to stop that unhealthy smoking habit for good. Finally, you can do away with smoking in 7 days if you want to. Yes, you can stop smoking in 7days with NO replacements, excessive weight gain or extra expenses. Rather you smoke seven cigarettes a day or seventy, you can stop smoking for good. This painless and fat-free habit kicking formula will free you from the chains of smoking without the weight gain. Furthermore, this stop smoking 7days guide will free you from smoking without any ongoing substitutions or expensive drug replacement aids whatsoever. I will not allude to any magical trick or false accusation as to how easy it is to stop a habit that possible has been part of your life for numerous years, or decades. I will assure you, what will make this entire program doable is desire and confidence. A strong desire accompanied by confident expectation of its fulfillment will accomplish much.

Please, once and for all let us lay to rest all the nonsense about smoking and expensive scientific research. Let us lay to rest all the drug replacement junk and advertising claims we see on Television. You can apply this technique not only to smoking, but also to any habit that you feel you would like to alter.

Please note: If you do not want to sincerely stop smoking-nothing is going to help you. No drug, No patch, No amount to food consumption, complaints or even death will end your desire to be smoke. We will feed our desires whatever they may be or consequences they hold.

The best part about this 7day guide is you can't fail. If, for some reason, you fail at your first attempt, start over again. You can restart this program at any time and as often as you like. There are no losers and no limits. Kicks start this program until you are totally successful.

About the author

On a personal note, **an informed smoker is a former smoker.** I too was a hard-core smoker. I smoked a pack of cigarettes a day for numerous years. Being with child or born with a serious heart defect did not prevent me from smoking for a very long time. As if smoking with a congenital heart defect was not serious enough, I started smoking at a very early age, as a punk kid. Weirdly reasonably I thought it made me look cool, while trying to fit in with the other kids. Unfortunately, I did not realize the consequence or observe the full picture in its entirety. Eventually, foolishness met up with reality, and I had to face the fact that my addiction was ruling and robbing the quality of my life. How strange, sometimes when we participate or indulge in certain activities we seem to be so far removed from our common sense.

Much too often we are so selfish or self-centered we fail to consider others that our addictions, or if you prefer the milder term habits' seriously effect. I smoked all through my teen years and throughout my pregnancy. Unfortunately, sometimes we can be rebellious and selfish and appear to focus only on ourselves. I am now smoke-free with nothing but remorse and a strong desire to help free others from this horrible smelly bondage called cigarette smoking.

If you care about yourself at all and care about your loved ones, quit smoking ASAP. You will like yourself more, and you and your loved ones will live much longer.

What exactly is smoking?

Smoking is one of the most common forms of recreational drug use. Smoking releases the addictive drug called nicotine that's inhaled through your nose and mouth through your lungs into your bloodstream.

Smoking is a form of a drug and has been around for many, many centuries – Yes; that's correct; it's a recreational drug!

There are so many products advertised on the market claiming to free you from your smoking addiction- Not only do they not work, but many risk becoming addicted to the very product that claims to help free you.

I don't know about you, but I am sick and tired of the drug pushing commercials. Are you as sick and tired of the insanity of using drugs to overcome things that are in our own self-control as I am? How hypocritical is it drug trafficking is declared illegal yet every other commercial on public television is pushing drugs on individuals all over America in other forms? (Prescription drugs)

Quiz

Take this quick quiz and find out if you might have a smoking habit?

Am I addicted?

1, Do you look forward to the opportunity to light up a cigarette?

2, Have you ever sneaked and smoked when and where it's prohibited?

3, Do it offend you or upset you when you are asked not to smoke?

4, Do you continued to smoke even when faced with a health problem that is directly caused by or worsened by smoking?

5, Have you ever smoked in the car or home of a non smoker who may be harmed by your smoke?

6, Are you willing to give up or reduce the number of work-related, recreational, or social activities for the sake of smoking

7, Have you tried to quit smoking and failed?

8, Do you anticipate smoking a cigarette after spending a great deal of time in activity or when smoking was not allowed? (Such as air travel, class, etc...)

9, Have you developed a tolerance to nicotine requiring greater amounts at times?

10, Do you suffer withdrawal symptoms when you attempt to stop smoking?

Quiz Evaluation

How many questions did you answer yes to? If you answered yes to over four, you have a smoking habit. Good news, you can break it if you set your mind on eliminating your intake of smoke.

Q&A

Q. Does smoking make me look attractive or cool?
A. Smoking is not only dangerous to you and all within breathing distance, but also ages you quicker and embeds a horrible lingering order onto your clothing, hair and breath.   How attractive is that?

Q, Is smoking really as bad for me as the warnings claim it is?
A. Yes, smoking is not only dangerous to but you everyone around you as well.

Q. What other effect can smoking have on the smoker?
A. According to WebMD, there maybe no fountain of youth, but there is a surefire way to make yourself look older. Smoking changes the skin, teeth, and hair in ways that can add years to your looks. It also affects everything from your fertility to the strength of your heart, lungs, and bones.

Q. How is my cigarette smoking harmful to those around me?
A. According to the Mayo Clinic, exposure to the toxins in secondhand smoke can cause asthma, cancer and other serious problems. When you decide to smoke, you make a decision for everyone around you to smoke, including children.

Q. What benefits will I gain from quitting smoking?
A. If finances are more important to you than your health, do the math. If you care at all about your health and your loved ones, you will save yourself from heart and lung

disease, other major health issues from quitting. You will all live and love much longer.

Stop Smoking 7 Days

Come on, admit it, you enjoy a cigarette with coffee, after dinner or on that drive to work; I did! Smoking is one of those love-hate relationships that many of us get ourselves into. Smoking or any other habit that grows and grows and must be cut off at the root. Bad habits seem easy enough to form that a child can do it. Bad habits are sometimes difficult for an adult to alter or break because of the effort we put into building and strengthening the behavior.

Addiction – Characteristic mode of growth or occurrence.
Habit - Any repetitive behavior pattern forms a habit.
Habit has several definitions according to the Merriam dictionary:

1, Clothing –
2, Manner of conducting ones self –
3, A settled tendency or usual manner of behavior-
4, A behavior pattern acquired by frequent repetition or physiologic exposure that shows itself in regularity or increased facility of performance –
5, An acquired mode of behavior that has become nearly or completely involuntary

Please read the above definitions again slowly and meditate upon them searching out the common dominator. You should have drawn the conclusion that the common dominator is: an addictive behavior pattern enforced by repetition.

It's never easy to break a bad habit, but possible.

History of Smoking –

You might be surprised that over one billion people practice tobacco smoking. It is by far the most popular form of smoking in the majority of all human societies.

The history of smoking can be dated as early as 5000 BC, and has been recorded in many different cultures across the world. In Europe, smoking introduced a new type of social activity and a form of drug intake, which previously had been unknown. The practice of smoking tobacco quickly spread to the rest of the world after the European exploration and conquest of the Americans. Ref: Merriam dictionary.

Danger of smoking

Cigarette smoking causes numerous Deaths by inhaling the smoke to the smoker. Cigarette smoking causes death to those around you through your second-hand smoke. Medical studies have proven that smoking tobacco is among the leading causes of many diseases such as lung cancer, heart attacks, COPD, Erectile dysfunction and can also lead to birth defects.

Dangers of smoking according to the American Cancer Society.

- **Your health**

Smoking harms nearly every organ of the human body. Half of all smokers who continue to smoke end up dying from smoke-related illiness. Smoking is responsible for nearly 1 in five deaths in the USA. Alone. About, 8.6

million people suffer from smoking-related lung and heart diseases.

- **Cancer**

Most of us realize that smoking can cause lung cancer, but few people realize it is also linked to higher risk for many other kinds of cancer too, including cancer of the mouth, nose, sinuses, voice box (larynx), throat (pharynx), esophagus, bladder, kidney, pancreas, ovary, cervix, stomach, colon, rectum, and acute myeloid leukemia.

- **Lung diseases**

According to the American cancer society - Smoking greatly increases your risk of getting long-term lung diseases like emphysema and chronic bronchitis. These diseases make it harder to breathe, and are grouped together under the name *chronic obstructive pulmonary disease* (COPD). COPD causes chronic illness and disability, and gets worse over time – sometimes becoming fatal. Emphysema and chronic bronchitis can be found in people as young as 40, but are usually found later in life, when the symptoms become much worse. Long-term smokers have the highest risk of developing severe COPD. Pneumonia is also included in the list of diseases caused or made worse by smoking.

- **Heart attacks, strokes, and blood vessel diseases**

Smokers are twice as likely to die from heart attacks as non-smokers. Smoking is a major risk factor for *peripheral vascular disease*, a narrowing of the blood vessels that carry blood to the leg and arm muscles. Smoking also affects the walls of the vessels that carry blood to the brain (carotid arteries), which can cause strokes. Smoking can cause *abdominal aortic aneurysm*, in which the layered walls of the body's main artery (the aorta) weaken and separate, often causing sudden death. And men who smoke are more likely to develop Erectile dysfunction (impotence) because of blood vessel disease.

- **Special risks to women and babies**

Women have some unique risks linked to smoking. Women over 35 who smoke and use birth control pills have a higher risk of heart attack, stroke, and blood clots in the legs. Women who smoke are more likely to miscarry (lose the baby) or have a lower birth-weight baby. And low birth-weight babies are more likely to die, or have learning and physical problems.

Benefits to quitting smoking According to the American Cancer Society.

No matter how old you are or how long you've smoked, quitting can help you live longer and be healthier. Quitting smoking has major and immediate health benefits for men and women of all ages. These benefits apply to people who already have smoking-related diseases and those who don't.

Ex-smokers live longer than people who keep smoking.

Giving up cigarette smoking is one of the most difficult tasks anyone can do during their life. Although numerous smokers have inhaled through their last breath, millions have been successful at kicking the nasty habit of cigarette smoking and have a greater chance of enjoying a longer life span. Some smokers have made several unsuccessful attempts to quit but refuse to give up, eventually are successful and enjoy living a smoke-free life.

Additional Benefits of Quitting Smoking- according to your household.

Let's not forget the cost of a pack of cigarettes today. You do the math and conclude how much you contribute to the tobacco institution. I'm sure you have much better places you could distribute weekly financial consumption used on dangerous smoke.

More Benefits of Quitting Smoking – according to your family and co inhabits

You and your co inhabits will live longer, look and feel better and definitly smell better.

Everyone will benefit from you living a smoke free life.

Good News

Rather, your smoking intake consists of seven cigarettes a day or seventy; YOU <u>CAN</u> stop smoking for good. Cigarette smoking is nothing more than a habitual daily pattern that you can alter. You can overcome any obstacle in life, including years of smoking.

Bad News -

If you refuse to stop smoking, eventually you will suffer consequences in one way or another - The toxic smoke will eventually take your life or the life of a loved one who falls victim to your second hand smoke.

About this book and program

This book consists of a 7day program. I must warn you that the first day /first step is the most difficult. Once you conquer day one the rest will be a cinch. Fear not, I will walk you through the entire program over and over if need be. I'm totally confident that you will master this, and be celebrating your smoke-free life in just 7 days or shortly thereafter.

If you have played any interactive video game, you understand the strategic levels to conquer, before you win the game. This quit smoking technique is closely related or likened unto an interactive video game. Once you become familiar with the game, the game becomes easier.

Step one –

On paper, map out your general daily routine and pinpoint all of your smoking rituals. E.g.-with coffee, commuting, after dinner, after sex, during conversation, drinking, movie intermission, etc. Keep this ritual smoking map aside for your reference.

1. Add up how many times daily you smoke a cigarette?
2. Take note -which area or at what time you smoke most frequently?
3. Being perfectly honest with yourself will help you the most.

Remember these two things.
1. You can do this; you can do away with smoking if you want to. Yes, you too can stop smoking in 7days with NO replacements, no extra weight gain or nicotine replacement products.
2. If you sincerely do not want to stop smoking- Nothing is going to help you. No drug, No patch, No amount to food consumption, complaints or even death will end your desire to be smoke. We will feed our desires whatever they may be or consequences they hold.

Again, the best part about this 7day guide is you can't fail. If, for some reason, you mess us, you simply start over again and again if need be until you are totally successful.

Now, decide on a stop-smoking date that you are sincere about and let's get started.

Day One:

Congratulations, you have made a very wise decision. Today is the first day of enjoying the rest of your life.

This is a 7day 7step program. I'm totally confidant you will master this and be celebrating your smoke-free life in just 7 days or shortly thereafter.

Start this day out with (7) Cigarettes…. A good and positive attitude will keep you strong all day. Please try to smoke only these cigarettes for the entire day- DO NOT RESEVE ANY PART OF THESE FOR LATER USE! Most smokers are guilty of salvaging cigarette butts… ☹ Please do not do this!
Saving any portion of these cigarettes for later use will ruin your journey to success.

 You only have seven cigarettes for the entire day, so use them wisely. Again, very important Note: Do not save any portion for later use…

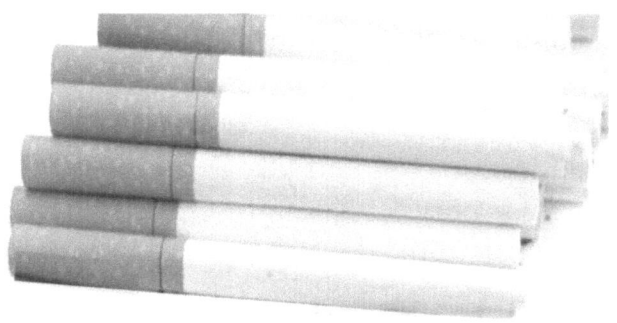

The most important accomplishment we are after on day one of this smoking program is a process of elimination. We want to pinpoint your heaviest smoking rituals first and eliminate them.

Closely observe your daily smoking pattern that you created or jotted down earlier in step one and number them one to seven. Number them according to your greatest urge to smoke – The greatest being first down to the very least. Let's start with number one, the most troubled cigarette smoking ritual– e.g., Coffee time, drive to work, your commute to and from home, etc.. Eliminating this area first will make the rest of the program a breeze to conquer.

Before anyone can break a habit, there are obstacles we must do away with before we reach your goal. Breaking the link between smoking and the activity that it's related to will also break the chains of bondage of any habit. It's nothing more than good ole common sense; breaking a ritual will break the habit. If we are in the ritual habit of smoking every time we close our car door we must break that particular ritual. Let's say instead of lighting a cigarette, insert a ticktack, breath mint or cough drop to put in your mouth. Doing something other than our usual smoking will break this ritual. We only have to do this until we become accustomed to your new smoke free commuting.

A personal suggestion, I would talk to God. Thank him for all his blessings or pray for strength, my children or loved one's safety and salvation.

Note: Do not substitute with food or other unhealthy habit-forming rituals.

If you were successful at day one, congratulations, your achievement will greatly pay off physically, financially and spiritually. If you were not totally successful, do not fret, as I said earlier, with this 7day program, you cannot fail. Like playing that interactive video game, simply start over. Star over as if it were the first-day – over and over again if need be!

Day Two

Congratulations, you have made it through day one and step one. As I forewarned you, day one was the hardest.

Start this day, day (2) out with Six Cigarettes and a good winning positive attitude. Please try to smoke only these cigarettes for the entire day- DO NOT RESEVE ANY PART OF THESE FOR LATER USE! All smokers are guilty of salvaging cigarette butts… ☹

You only have six cigarettes for the entire day, so use them wisely.

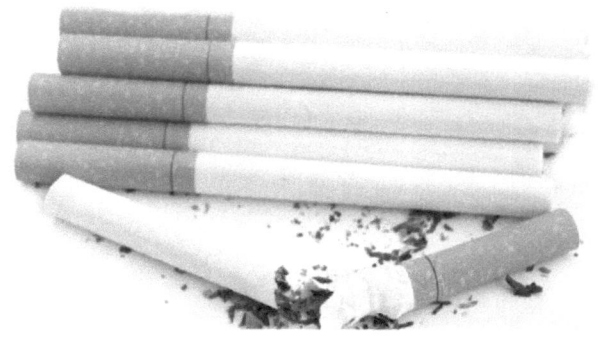

Very important Note: Do not save any portion for later use…

Day one should be marked as complete on your frequently list. With day one accomplished, take a quick look at day two on your daily smoking pattern map. Now, work earnestly, and with a good positive attitude on tackling number two from your daily smoking rituals. We are after

26

the same eliminating process as day one of your most frequently smoking urge. Let's say number two is a 15-minute smoking break at work, or smoking while talking on the phone. Try skipping at least one of your 10 -15 minute smoking breaks or avoid the phone all together if possible. If you must take the phone call, try doodling or something instead of lighting up that cigarette.

Important Note: Do not substitute with food or other unhealthy habit-forming rituals.

Keeping abreast, the most powerful accomplishment we are after in this 7-day program is eliminating the frequent troublesome smoking areas first – 1 though 7

Day Three -

Congratulations, you have made it through one and day two of our 7day stop smoking program! You are almost half way through, you should be very proud of yourself-you have done well.

With day two accomplished, take a quick look at day three on your smoking pattern map. It's now time to eliminate day (3). Start day three out with Five (5) whole Cigarettes and a good winning positive attitude. Please try to smoke only these cigarettes for the entire day- A friendly reminder - ☺ -most smokers are guilty of salvaging cigarette butts for later use, please do not do this.

You only have five cigarettes for the entire day, so use them wisely. If you were successful at day one and two, your smoking should be down to 5 cigarettes daily. If you feel you were not all that successful, please keep trying. If you keep the faith and the desire to stop smoking, you will be successful.

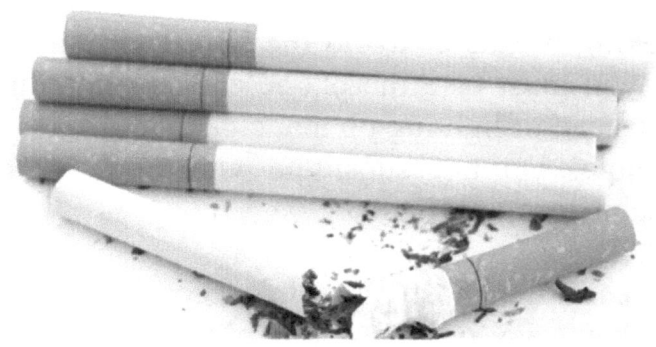

Very important Note: Do not save any portion for later use...

Now, work earnestly, and with a good positive attitude on eliminating number three from your daily smoking rituals. We are after the same eliminating process as day one, and day two of your most frequently smoking urge. Let's say number three on your daily smoking ritual takes place after meals. Try sipping a bottle or glass of water with several drops of fresh lemon juice. Sipping lemon water has helped stop many bad habits, from smoking to soda pop consumption; I know this first hand. Not too long ago I was addicted to drinking several cans of soda pop a day. Now, thanks to lemon water, I maybe have one?
Rather, my suggestions work for you, or you have your own ideas; you must somewhat personalize this program to fit you. This program is designed to make you aware of your smoking habitual pattern. It's designed to inform you;

you must eliminate the rituals in order to eliminate the habit.

Important Note: Do not substitute your smoking cigarettes with food or other unhealthy habit-forming rituals.

Keep abreast, the most powerful accomplishment we are after in this 7-day program is eliminating the frequent troublesome smoking areas first – 1 though 7

Day Four

WOW, you've come a long way from the health-damaging smoker you were just several days ago. Way to go! You should be very proud of yourself and feeling better already. You have done well.

With day three behind you, look at number four on your smoking pattern map. It's now time to eliminate number (4) from your daily life. Let's earnestly work hard today at eliminating all but 4 cigarettes from your life. Rather, you smoke 4 cigarettes a day or a pack of 20; your health is at risk from the harmful chemicals contained in tobacco. Start day four with Four (4) cigarettes and a good positive attitude. Please try to smoke only these cigarettes for the entire day- Please do not salvage any part of today's cigarette for later use. ☺

You only have four cigarettes for the entire day, use them wisely. If you were successful at day one, two and three, your smoking should be down to 4 cigarettes for the day. If you were not successful in the previous days, please keep trying. Again, if you keep the faith and the desire to stop smoking, you will be successful.

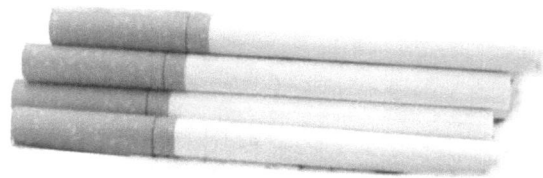

Very important Note: Do not save any portion for later use…

If you are in good health, shame on you for actively and deliberately destroying your health. When in good health, we should be thanking God for our health, and not destroying it. There are millions of people who would be extremely grateful to be in good health. If you are in poor health, exactly what do you think inhaling harmful carbon monoxide, cyanide, and other chemicals will benefit you? Just saying! Keeping a good and positive attitude, with a constant reminder of all the negative harmful effects smoking holds will carry a great amount of influence on your desire to quit.

Nearing the end of your list number four smoking ritual should be less important and easier to eliminate than your number one. Number four on your list, maybe a cigarette you could avoid altogether, without any thought or very little emphases on it whatsoever. We are after the same eliminating process as day one, day two and day three of your most frequently smoking urges. If you need to occupy or substitute, try sipping a bottle or glass of lemon water, sucking on a menthol cough drop.

Important Note: Do not substitute your smoking cigarettes with food or other unhealthy habit-forming rituals. Rather, my suggestions work for you, or you have your own ideas; you must somewhat personalize this program to fit you. This program is to inform you; you must eliminate the rituals in order to eliminate the habit.

Day Five

OK, I expect you have already started enjoying the extra breath and freedom from the bondage of cigarette smoking? You have probably already begun to pass the word on about this program? ☺

I am very confidant you have gotten through this and looking forward to the last day of the program. You have come a long way, and I'm proud of you. I'm not going to arrogantly tell you it's easy to quit smoking; it's not, but it's crucial.

Look at number 5 on your smoking pattern map. It's now time to eliminate this number (5) from your daily life as well. If you have successfully followed this program, you should be down to only three cigarettes a day. If, for some reason, you have not been successful at following along with this program, you can begin again or wherever you fell short. You can follow this program over and over again. Whatever you do, never give up or stop trying to conquer a bad habit.

With numbers one, two, three and four removed from your list, you should be able to see the light at the end of the tunnel. Seeing a light at the end of our tunnel does in no way mean it is easier, but is possible.

Start day 5 out with only 3 cigarettes.

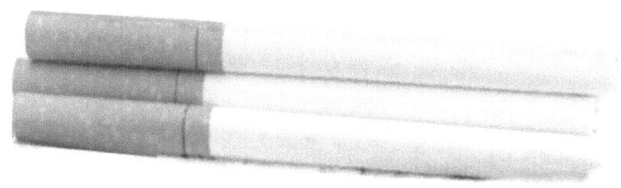

You only have three cigarettes for the entire day, use them wisely. Please do not reserve any part of these cigarettes for later use, it will null and void the impact of this program. Number three-cigarette ritual may be after the kids go to bed, after long or short nonsmoking journey, checking emails, etc.? Putting an end to this smoking ritual will not require avoiding this time only find a soothing alternate. Might I suggest a nice hot cup of soothing green tea, or reading a few scriptures? Whatever you choose as an alternative, you must choose wisely. Imperative you don't replace one bad habit with another habit that is equally as harmful to your health and those around you. If successful at day one, two, three and four, the next part of your smoking habit should be a breeze to overcome?

You are so close to the end of this journey now you can start celebrating, ☺

Let's savor your successful steps with a nice bottle of water and some thanksgiving. You can now add up your savings you will benefit from for the rest of your life. You will grow to appreciate all the smokeless days more and more as the days and years go by. You will be pleased you decided to take this stop-smoking journey.

Day Six

About this time in the program, I'm more than excited for your success. We are all but finished with this program that we journey together, and I cannot wait to hear your story. At the end of the book I am going to include a contact address to submit all success stories. But for now, lets continue and complete our 7day stop smoking program. We have reached day 6, and only one step away from home base. Day six of most journeys are dreadful, but with this program, day six should be a day of rejoicing.

Start day (6) out with only 2 cigarettes.

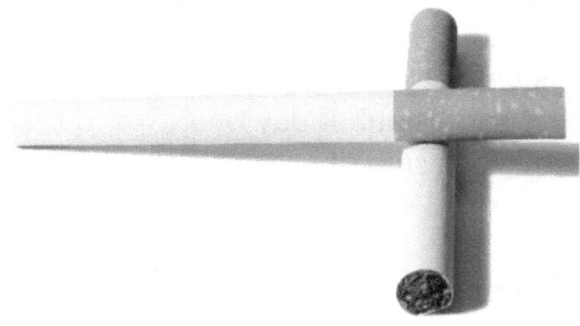

You only have two cigarettes for the entire day, use them wisely. Vital, please do not reserve any part of these two cigarettes for later use. Reserving a portion of these two cigarettes will totally ruin the success of your journey thus far. These two cigarette rituals may be a time killer, (latterly), just because, or before bed, etc... At this point, in your journey, you have already determined to finish or decided you like smoking and will continue? I'm going to give you the benefit and continue on as if you are following along with. These two cigarettes, treat with utmost respect and value. Treasure these two cigarettes as a child who treasures his or her bottle at nap-time. Smoke one of these cigarettes in the morning and save the last until night… Anytime, you get the urge to smoke during the day, anticipate or focus on smoking that last cigarette before bed.

Note: always try to substitute or counteract your urge to smoke with a healthy alternative. Avoid interchanging one bad habit for another damaging substance.

Day Seven

WOW! Congratulations, you have now reached the end of our stop smoking in 7day program. You have now truly earned bragging rights. ⓑⓡ I'm praying you have sailed through this journey with excitement and expectation. After all, your success is my success. If you happened to falter, please keep on keeping on.

We are on the last day and finished with this stop smoking program that we journey together 7days ago.

Today your daily smoking list should be all crossed off with last step remaining. I'm sure by now, the last day of our journey; you figured out the pattern? Start this day out with (1) cigarette?

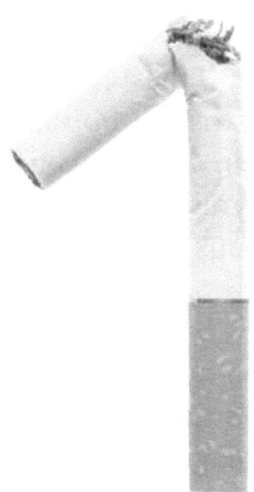

After creating your daily smoking ritual, and prioritizing them from 1 to 7, one being most smoked, what stronghold could number 7 possibly have over you? NONE! Congratulations again… You're awesome!

The best thing about this program, besides living a smoke-free life, is realizing you don't need it. It's a throw away. I too was a smoker from a very early age… I did it and so can you…. Never give up….

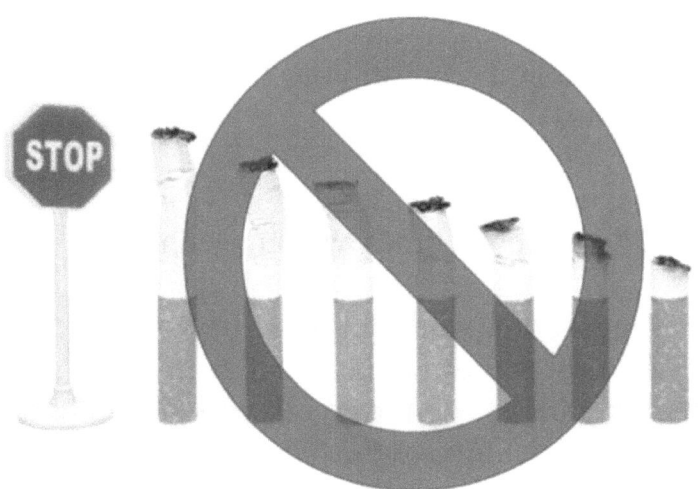

You have successfully Kicked this nasty habbit

Living Smoke Free, what now?

Be careful not to entertain or dabble with this dangerous smoking habit ever again. Smoking is like being an alcoholic; you cannot walk away with just one drink.

Make it your mission to help others to kick the habit of cigarette smoking.

Try avoiding times that make you vulnerable to lighting up a cigarette. Try to avoid smoking areas and gatherings. Find a soothing alternate such as, a nice hot cup of soothing green tea, or reading a few scriptures? Whatever you choose as an alternative, you must choose wisely.

Failed attempts:

Never allow any habit to control your life, but let your life control your habits.

You can do this; never give up….
Try it repeatedly, as many times as you need to.

Rather, my suggestions work for you, or you have your own ideas; you must somewhat personalize this program to fit you. This program is to inform you; you must eliminate the rituals in order to eliminate the habit.

Try avoiding times that make you vulnerable to lighting up a cigarette. Try to avoid smoking areas and gatherings. Find a soothing alternate such as, a nice hot cup of soothing green tea, or reading a few scriptures? Whatever you choose as an alternative, you must choose wisely.

Note: always try to substitute or counteract your urge to smoke with a healthy alternative. Avoid interchanging one bad habit for another damaging substance that could become part of your life or your loved one's life.

Q&A

Q. What if I fail at this program?
A. Try again, and again, and again if need to. There is absolutely no pressure or limit to the times you can try.

Q. Can I use this book to help other smokers?
A. Absolutely, we encourage it… you may give your purchased copy away or resell it, but it is copyright material; you cannot copy and resell this program in any deliverable form.

Q. Why do you always suggest prayer or mediation?
A. Prayer has never harmed anyone, but the lack there of has. We would do well to pray about everything in our lives. Maybe including prayer in our daily life, we would pick up fewer bad habits and more of the good?

Q. Why does this book consist of such redundancy?
A. Redundancy helped get us into bad habits; it can help get us out. You can never be encouraged enough.

Q. Is harshness or scolding really necessary?
A. Often times, constructive criticism can be a valuable tool.

Send us your success story.

Visit our web site www.stopsmoking7days.info
Refer others to us… www.stopsmoking7days.info

Other books. – Author Becky Gruber
www.beckybooks.com

Created with purpose –
God's Toolbox-

Loan Origination
Without a Vision, People Perish
Life's missing piece
Christian 101

Great books from other authors –
How to become a dental assistant without a degree or
experience –
Sheila Schiff - www.dentalassistantopportunity.com

Loan Officer training
Building Teen Character
Loan Processing Training

Available for purchase –

www.purposelife.info - www.Amazon.com –
http://www.barnesandnoble.com/w/created-with-purpose-
bargainhouse-publication/1019607880 - www.lulu.com -
http://www.smashwords.com/books/view/26937

Notes: